Homemade Body Butters

Simple Recipes for Soft, Healthy, and Beautiful Looking Skin. Rejuvenate your Skin Naturally!

Jane Moore

Contents

Introduction

Your Skin and You

Making Your Own Body Butter

   The Secret to Making Your Body Butter

52 Body Butter Recipes

   #1 Peppermint & Citrus Whipped Body Butter

   #2 Vanilla Bean Body Butter

   #3 Key Lime Whipped Coconut Oil Body Butter

   #4 Mint Chocolate Whipped Body Butter

   #5 Peppermint and Shea Butter Body Butter

   #6 Bronzer Whipped Body Butter

   #7 Rosemary Tea Tree Body Butter

   #8 Shea and Coconut Body Butter

   #9 Whipped Peppermint Tallow Body Butter

   #10 Anti Bacterial Body Butter

   #11 Sweet Almond Body Butter Recipe

   #12 Magnesium Body Butter

   #13 The "To Die For" Body Butter

   #14 Buff Body Butter

   #15 Simple Moisturizing Body Butter

   #16 Jojoba and Shea Butter Whipped Body Butter

   #17 Jojoba and Lavender Relaxing Body Butter

   #18 Jojoba and Peppermint Refreshing Body Butter

   #19 Lavender Body Butter

   #20 Rosemary Mint Whipped Shea Body Butter

   #21 Mango Citrus Body Butter

#22 Coconut Rose Body Butter

#23 Almond Body Butter

#24 Super Glowy Jasmine Body Butter

#25 Whipped Argan & Mango Body Butter

#26 Cinnamon Body Butter for Cellulite

#27 Chocolate Body Butter Recipe

#28 Coffee Butter Foot Cream

#29 Dreamy Homemade Lemon Cream Body Butter Recipe

#30 Decadent Whipped Body Butter

#31 Pretty in Pink Body Butter

#32 Homemade Coconut Vanilla Body Butter

#33 Honey and Lemon Body Butter

#34 Eczema Fighting Body Butter

#35 Christmas Mango and Mint Body Butter

#36 Coconut & Plum Whipped Body Butter

#37 Orange & Coconut Whipped Body Butter

#38 Eucalyptus Mint Whipped Body Butter

#39 Wild Orange Body Butter Recipe

#40 Honey Kissed Massage Body Butter

#41 Aromatherapy Lavender & Rose Flower Body Butter

#42 Aromatherapy Lavender Spice Body Butter

#43 Varicose Vein Attacking Body Butter

#44 Tangerine Whipped Body Butter

#45 Mountain Rose Herb Body Butter

#46 Mint Chocolate Whipped Body Butter

#47 Whipped Peppermint Bark Body Butter

#48 Calming Orange Vanilla Whipped Body Butter

#49 Cranberry Body Butter Whip

#50 Sugar Cookie Body Butter

#51 Strawberry Body Butter

#51 Avocado Body Butter

#52 Lavender and Lace Body Butter

Main Ingredients Explained

Shea Butter

Mango

Coconut Oil

Lavender

Cocoa

Kokum or Illipe Butters

Almond

Mandarin

Olive Oil

Hemp Oil

Coffee Bean, Macadamia, Pistachio

Aloe Vera

Jojoba Oil

Tallow

Vitamin E

Essential Oils

Waxes

Beeswax

Candelilla Wax

CO2 Extracts

Attars

Fragrance Oils

Additives

Cornstarch

Silk Powder

Antioxidants

Basic Recipes for Whipped Body Butters

Basic Whipped Shea Butter

Basic Whipped Hard Butter

Basic Whipped Medium-Soft Butter

Basic Whipped Solid Oil

Basic Whipped Soft-Butter

How to Buy Essential Oils

Organic Essential Oils

Tips

Conclusion

Introduction

As winter approaches, the sound of a crackling fire comes to mind, with warm air circulating throughout the house. However, for many of us, with that comes dry skin that can be a real problem. Then again dealing with dry skin doesn't have to be a 'winter' thing. Some of us deal with dry skin in the dry heat or all the time with no relation to the weather.

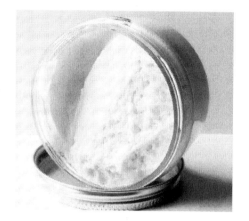

Whatever your reason for dry skin that need tending to, chances are you've tried a number of different commercial products

Then again, it might not be dry skin – perhaps you are just looking to enjoy soft, supple, more youthful skin that's healthy looking. Chances are you've used commercial products.

Since you have this book in your hand, we can only assume that you are either not satisfied with the commercial products you've tried or you are looking for a more natural alternative.

Great news! You are not going to be disappointed. Here you are going to find all kinds of amazing homemade body butters to pamper your body and nourish it. These body butters will keep your skin smooth, supple, and moisturized.

Unlike the products you purchase at a store, the body butter you make contains fresh, nutritional ingredients with no chemicals or preservatives.

Best of all, it takes very little time to actually make your own body butter. It's easy and it's economical. We're going to give you tons of great recipes that have been made and tested so all you have to do is have some fun making them.

It's time to pamper yourself –you will feel like you've just been to a luxurious spa.

Your Skin and You

Did you know that your skin is your largest organ? Did you know that your skin absorbs many of the things that it comes in contact with whether these are bad or good? This is why some drugs are administered using a patch! It takes only 26 seconds for your skin to absorb any substance that you apply to it.

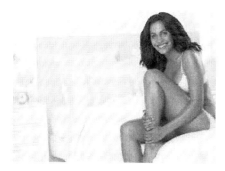 The problem is it is very difficult to find a commercial skin care product that is doesn't contain harmful chemicals. The majority of commercial products contain petroleum based chemicals, known carcinogens that are used as preservatives like BHT and titanium dioxide, and known hormone disruptors like parabens.

The majority of ingredients in these products are chemicals – if you can't pronounce the name, chances are it's not good for you. Even with natural and organic products you need to be careful and actually read the ingredients.

According to the Organic Consumer Association there is a great deal of misleading on the labeling for organics.

A newly released study commissioned by the Organic Consumers Association (OCA), a watchdog group with over 500,000 members, and overseen by environmental health consumer advocate David Steinman (author of The Safe Shopper's Bible*), analyzes leading "natural" and "organic" brand shampoos, body washes, lotions and other personal care products for the presence of the undisclosed carcinogenic contaminant 1,4-Dioxane. A reputable third-party laboratory known for rigorous testing and chain-of-custody protocols performed all testing.*

Visit any health food store unfortunately and you'll discover that the majority of products in the personal care section that are labeled 'organic' are not USDA-certified and contain only cheap water extracts of organic herbs and occasionally a handful of other organic ingredients as a token offer. The core of most of these products, including body lotions and moisturizers is composed of synthetic ingredients.

According to market statistics, consumers will pay significantly more for 'natural' or 'organic' products, because they believe they don't contain petrochemical ingredients or other toxic ingredients.

The good news is that it is very easy for you to make your own body butter and skin care products. When you make them yourself, you control the ingredients and you can ensure none of these toxic ingredients are in your product.

This book focuses on making your own body butter, but once you are comfortable making these products, why not branch out and try your hand at some of the other personal care products you use.

Making Your Own Body Butter

Don't be afraid. Making your own body butter is not any harder than making icing for your cake. The process is very similar and you already will likely have all of the tools in your kitchen.

Most body butters that you will make contain only a few ingredients like coconut oil, essential oils and tallow. It's great that you can make your body butter, whatever scent you desire and you can take advantage of the therapeutic qualities that some of the oils have. Let your imagination run wild – the sky is the limit!

If you are like so many of us you've spent hundreds of dollars on store bought lotions that you aren't happy with. Even a visit to your local health food store can be disappointed as you scour the shelves looking for a lotion that contains the ingredients you want. The solution is simple – make your own! Have fun and don't be afraid to experiment.

The Secret to Making Your Body Butter

Making your own body butter isn't difficult. It's really very simple to make, just follow the recipe. The key is to use the correct combination of solid and liquid oils so that you get a consistency that can be whipped just like you would do with soft butter that you were going to use to make a whipped cream icing.

These recipes are fresh without chemicals for preservatives so they are not going to last for years, but if you store them in the refrigerator in a glass jar that seals you'll extend their shelf life.

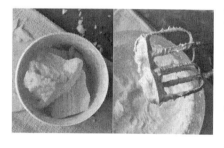 Do this unless the recipe gives another suggestion.

The glass canning jars, which come in a number of smaller sizes, are great for this. You can fancy them up with a pretty ribbon and they are easy to label.

One thing we should mention, rather than filling the pages with pictures of the steps of mixing and pouring, which we're pretty sure you can handle without a picture, we're going to use our page space to pack in as many body butter recipes as we can.

Our thought was you'd rather have more options than more pictures.

Are you ready? This book is packed with tons of great homemade body butter recipes. Don't be afraid to modify any one of the recipes any way you like. Experimenting is half the fun.

You can make a new one for every week of the year and then some. Don't be surprised if you start making them for gifts. Okay, let's get started.

52 Body Butter Recipes

Let's get started. It's time to delve into the many great homemade body butter recipes we have for you.

#1 Peppermint & Citrus Whipped Body Butter

This is an easy DIY body butter recipe that is great for all skin types.

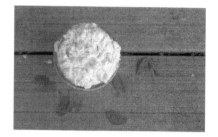

Ingredients:

- 1 cup Mango Butter
- 1 cup Coconut Oil
- 1 cup Shea Butter
- 1 cup light oil like olive or almond
- 10 drops of peppermint essential oil
- 30 drops of citrus essential oil

Instructions:

1. Take a double boiled and combine all or your ingredients, but not the essential oils.
2. On medium heat, let your ingredients melt while you constantly stir.
3. Remove from the heat and let it slightly cool.

4. Move the mixture to refrigerator and let cool for an hour or until you see it begin to harden slightly.

5. Use your hand mixer and whip for 10-15 minutes until it's fluffy.

6. Return to fridge for 10 to 15 minutes and let it set.

7. Place in glass jars with a lid to store.

8. Use as you would regular lotion or body butter.

9. If your home is 75 degrees or higher, it may become too soft. You can store it in the fridge.

Enjoy!

#2 Vanilla Bean Body Butter

This is an easy to make body butter that smells amazing and will deeply moisturize your skin, while at the same time soothing your soul.

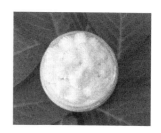

Ingredients:

- 2 cup raw cocoa butter
- 1 cup coconut oil
- 1 cup sweet almond oil
- 3 vanilla bean

Instructions:

1. In a double boiler, melt the cocoa butter and coconut oil over medium heat.
2. Once it is melted, remove from the heat and let cool for 30 minutes.
3. Grind your vanilla beans using your coffee grinder. You can also do this with a food processor.
4. Stir the sweet almond oil and vanilla bean bits into the cocoa butter and coconut oil.
5. Place it in the freezer for about 30 minutes to chill. Wait until oils start to partially solidify.

6. Whip with an electric mixer until it is butter-like consistency.
7. Spoon it into your glass jar(s). It makes about 5 cups of whipped butter. Store it in the refrigerator.

You'll feel sexy and sensual. Many cultures use this as an aphrodisiac; it's relaxing and pleasing to the mind, body and soul. You can apply it before bedtime to improve your sleep. Whip It: The Secret to Moisturizing with Coconut Oil

#3 Key Lime Whipped Coconut Oil Body Butter

This body butter smells so good you just might want to eat it. Delightful to apply all over and it also works great on those really dry spots like your elbows and heels. Give it a try.

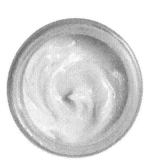

Ingredients:

- 1 cup coconut oil
- 2 tablespoon macadamia nut oil (or olive oil if you don't have macadamia nut)
- 4 tablespoons Aloe Vera gel
- 40 drops lime essential oil
- 40 drops lemon essential oil

Instructions:

1. Place all of your ingredients into a mixing bowl. Don't melt the coconut oil first because it has to be solid to whip up.
2. Use your electric mixer with a wire whisk. Put on high speed for 4 to 8 minutes or until it is whipped into a light, airy consistency.

3. Spoon the whipped coconut oil body butter into a glass jar and tightly cover.

4. Store at room temperature, unless your house is warm then refrigerate to prevent melting.

Smell your favorite dessert all the time!

#4 Mint Chocolate Whipped Body Butter

The is a great body butter for the hot season because it doesn't
melt too easily. Cocoa butter has a
higher melting point, which make
this body butter more stable during
the heat of summer.

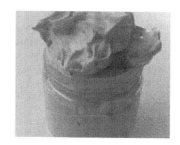

The peppermint oil in the whipped butter makes this refreshing
and cool in the summer heat.

Ingredients:
- 1 cup cocoa butter
- 1 cup coconut oil
- 40-60 drops peppermint essential oil

Instructions:
1. Add the cocoa butter and coconut into a double boiler.
2. On medium heat, stir constantly until they both have completely melted.
3. Cool the mixture in your refrigerator until it is mostly solid.
4. Sprinkle about 40 to 60 drops of peppermint essential oil on top – The amount of peppermint depends on how

strong you'd like the peppermint aroma and the cooling effect.

5. Every couple of minutes, stop your mixer and scrape the bowl sides. This will help to ensure it is mixed up really well so it's smoother.

6. Mix for appox. 10 minutes to get this body butter perfectly whipped and airy.

7. Scoop your mint chocolate whipped body butter into your glass jar and seal.

8. Store in the refrigerator.

#5 Peppermint and Shea Butter Body Butter

Peppermint is soothing and cooling. Add the Shea butter and it takes it to a whole new level. Experience it for yourself.

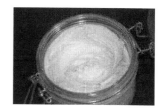

Ingredients:

- 2 cups of Shea butter
- 1 cup tallow
- 1 cup of jojoba oil
- 2 teaspoon peppermint essential oil
- 1 tablespoon Vitamin E oil

Instructions:

1. Use a double boiler to gently heat the Shea butter and tallow until they are completely melted.
2. Then remove the bowl from heat and stir in your Jojoba oil.
3. Set up an ice bath and let it chill for 5 minutes.
4. Stir in the peppermint essential oil and Vitamin E oil.
5. Let it keep chilling in the ice bath until it is thoroughly chilled.
6. Use your mixer to whip the butter mixture until it forms stiff peaks.

7. Scoop the mixture a put it into your glass jars and then seal. The Vitamin E is a natural preservative so when stored properly and away from direct sunlight, it should last for about 12 months.

#6 Bronzer Whipped Body Butter

This body butter smells so good, don't be surprised if you are

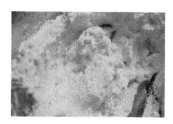

tempted to eat it – then again, it's no wonder with its great mix of cacao powder, nutmeg and cinnamon – yummy!

Eating it is perfectly harmless, but really it smells much better than it tastes, so just enjoy it on your body.

Ingredients:

- 1 cup coconut oil
- 1 cup Shea butter
- 1cup almond oil or jojoba oil
- 2-4 Tablespoons cocoa or cacao powder - You decide how dark your bronzer is by how much cacao powder you add. If you are fair skinned, a small amount is recommended.
- 2 Tablespoon ground nutmeg
- 4 Tablespoons ground cinnamon
- 2 teaspoons Vitamin E oil
- 10-15 drops of therapeutic essential oil

Instructions:

1. Using a double boiler and on low heat, melt your coconut oil on medium heat.
2. Once they are completely melted you can remove from the heat. Let stand to cool for 30 minutes.
3. Mix in the almond oil, cocoa/cacao powder, essential oil, cinnamon and nutmeg, Vitamin E.
4. Place the oil mixture in the freezer and let it firm up.
5. When the oil mixture is partially solidified, remove it you're your freezer and whip the mixture until it forms peaks. It should look like whipped butter.
6. Scoop into glass jars and seal.
7. The Vitamin E is a preservative so when stored properly out of direct sunlight, it should last 6 to 12 months.

Not only does this body butter smell terrific. You can choose therapeutic essential oils that can help you with an ailment such as inflammation or insomnia. In addition, you get the benefits of a natural bronzer to help your skin look great!

#7 Rosemary Tea Tree Body Butter

This body butter is perfect for those winter months when you need that additional moisturizing. The secret to making a

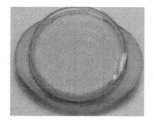

thicker butter is to use a ratio of 75% solid oil to 25% liquid oils or in other words a 3:1 ratio.

Ingredients:

- ¾ cup Shea butter
- 4 tablespoons cocoa butter
- ½ cup coconut oil
- ½ cup almond oil
- 25 drops rosemary essential oil
- 10 drops tea tree oil

Instructions:

1. In a double boiler on medium heat, melt your Shea butter, coconut oil and cocoa butter.
2. Remove from heat and let it cool for 30 minutes.
3. Once it has cooled, stir in your almond oil and essential oils.
4. Place the oil mixture in the refrigerator to cool for 15-25 minutes.

5. Check it regularly. When the outer edges of the mixture start to solidify, you need to whip the oils with your hand mixer until it turns into creamy body butter.

6. Place it in glass jars and seal. It will last for several months.

Tip: When whipping up this recipe it is very important to allow the oils to sufficiently cool before beginning the whipping process. If the oils are too warm they will not whip up to the creamy consistency you want.

#8 Shea and Coconut Body Butter

This body butter is a little greasy when you first put it on, but give it a few minutes and it will absorb, which is why it's best put on at night.

Ingredients:

- 1 cup Shea butter
- ½ cup coconut oil
- ½ cup almond oil (can substitute olive oil)
- 20-25 drops of your favorite essential oil

Instructions:

1. Combine all your ingredients into a double boiler.
2. Place over medium heat until everything is melted.
3. Pour into another bowl and let cool for at least an hour or until the oils are just starting solidify. If you want to speed it up you can place in the refrigerator.
4. When the oil mixture is starting to solidify around the edges, you can begin to beat with your mixer. Continue for 10-15 minutes, or until it begins to look something like whipped cream with the peaks forming.

5. Put into glass jars and seal. It should keep for quite some time as long as it is not stored in the direct sun or where it is too warm

Tips:

- Your measurements don't need to be exact. You can play with the consistency until you get what you like.
- It is important for it to be properly cooled for it to whip properly.

This body shows great results for very dry skin. Put it on at night and let it do its magic.

#9 Whipped Peppermint Tallow Body Butter

If you love peppermint, you are going to love this body, plus you can enjoy the benefits of tallow.

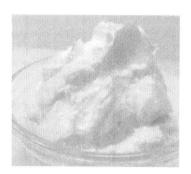

Ingredients:

- 2 cups of Shea butter
- 1 cup of jojoba oil
- 1 cup tallow
- 2 teaspoon peppermint essential oil
- 4 teaspoons vitamin E

Instructions:

1. Using a double boiler on medium heat, melt your Shea butter and tallow.
2. Remove your bowl from the heat and stir in your Jojoba oil.
3. Allow the mixture to chill in an ice bath for 5-10 minutes.
4. Then stir in the peppermint essential oil and Vitamin E oil.
5. Let the mixture continue to chill in the ice bath until it is thoroughly chilled.

6. Take your mixer and whip the body butter until it is stiff and forms peaks.
7. Place in glass jars and seal. Store away from direct sunlight. If you store it should keep about 1 year.

#10 Anti Bacterial Body Butter

This is one of those nice simple recipes and it's also anti bacterial an added bonus.

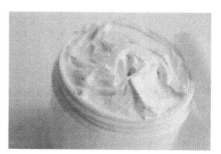

Ingredients:

- 1 cup coconut oil
- ½ cup cocoa butter
- 4 tablespoons Jojoba oil
- 1 teaspoon Vitamin E
- 20-25 drops of tea tree oil
- 15-20 drops of lavender or orange essential oil (optional)

Instructions:

1. Melt the cocoa butter in a double boiler on the stove top on low heat. You just want it dissolved, not hot.
2. When your cocoa butter has melted, remove it from heat and stir in your coconut oil, Jojoba oil and then combine the coconut oil, which should melt from the cocoa butter temperature.
3. Wait a few hours until your mixture solidifies at room temperature. If you want to speed things up, you can put it in the refrigerator.

4. Take your mixer and whip on high for 5 to 10 minutes, stopping occasionally to stir down the sides when necessary.
5. Add in your tea tree oil and give it one last mix.

Tip:

- You can add more tea tree. At the strength in this recipe, it is still quite gentle so you should be able to use on sensitive skin, although you should always do a skin test.
- Many people do not like the medicinal smell of tea tree, which is why the optional essential oils in this recipe.

This decadent body butter is gentle enough for even the most sensitive areas of your body, and it is helpful on your shaven areas, feet and underarms.

#11 Sweet Almond Body Butter Recipe

Ingredients:

- 2 cup cocoa butter
- 1 cup coconut oil
- 1 cup sweet almond oil

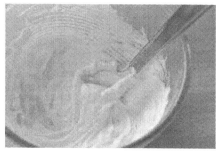

Instructions:

1. In a double boiler on medium heat, melt down your hard butters and oils until they are completely melted.
2. Set in the freezer for about 20 minutes to harden.
3. Once the mixture has started to solidify, but before it gets too hard, use your mixer to whip it until you have created fluffy peaks.
4. Spoon it into a glass jar and seal. It will keep for months.

#12 Magnesium Body Butter

This is a simple body butter that is created using simple ingredients while providing a soothing magnesium boost that will leave your skin silky and smooth.

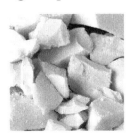

Ingredients:

- 1 cup Magnesium Flakes + 6 tablespoons boiling water or 1 cup of pre-made magnesium oil
- ½ cup unrefined coconut oil
- 4 tablespoons Beeswax Pastilles
- 6 tablespoons Shea Butter

Instructions:

1. In a small container, pour 6 tablespoons of boiling water into your magnesium flakes and stir until they are dissolved.
2. You will be left with a thick liquid. Set aside to cool.
3. In a quart size Mason jar inside a small pan with 1 inch of water on medium heat, add the beeswax, Shea butter and coconut oil.
4. Once it is melted, remove the jar from the pan and let the mixture cool until it is room temp and slightly opaque.

5. Put it into a medium size bowl.

6. Use your mixer to blend the oil mixture.

7. Slowly, one drop at a time, add the dissolved magnesium mixture to the oil mixture while continuing to blend until all of the magnesium is added and your mixture is well mixed.

8. Stick in the refrigerator for 20 to 25 minutes.

9. Re-blend until you get the body butter consistency you desire.

10. Store in refrigerator for a cooling lotion or at room temp for up to two months.

This is a great body butter that not only leaves your body smooth and silky, but also healthier.

#13 The "To Die For" Body Butter

Ingredients:

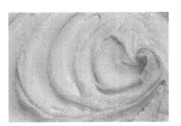

- 2 tablespoon mint infused coconut oil
- 2 tablespoon olive oil
- Dried rose petals
- Fresh rosemary or substitute another favorite herb
- 2 capsule Vitamin E
- 15 drops each of lime essential oil
- 20 drops lavender essential oil

Instructions:

1. The coconut oil you use can be solid or runny; it's all the same, just try to find some unrefined coconut oil/fat.
2. Melt your Shea butter and coconut oil in a double boiler on medium heat.
3. Add in the vegetable oil and if then your rosemary and rose petals.
4. Heat the herb mixture for about 25-30 minutes, then strain squeeze out the last of the oil from the herbs.
5. Remove from heat, and let cool.
6. When the mixture is 30C or cooler, add the essential oils and Vitamin E.

7. Whip the butter until it gets thick and fluffy. This will take 5 to 15 minutes. If it doesn't seem to be forming peaks let the batch cool a little longer until it's starting to solidify, then try again.

8. Spoon into glass jars and seal.

Tips:

- You can leave out the Vitamin E if you like, but it extends the shelf life and it is excellent for dry skin.
- To reduce costs, you can substitute any vegetable oil for the olive oil.
- If you want a really divine body butter substitute Jojoba, apricot or avocado oil for the olive oil.
- You can change the essential oils to your favorites.
- You can substitute your favorite herb(s) for the rosemary.

#14 Buff Body Butter

Ingredients:

- 6 ounces Shea butter
- 6 ounces cocoa butter
- 30 drops lemon essential oils
- 30 drops lavender essential oils
- ½ cup ground rice
- ¼ cup ground almonds
- Silicone small muffin molds

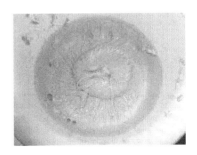

Instructions:

1. Measure out your Shea butter and cocoa butter into double boiler.
2. Place on medium heat until oil melts. The cocoa butter is hard so it will take a bit to melt.
3. While this is melting you can grind your rice and almonds in your food processor.
4. Once the oils are melted, add the essential oils, rice and almonds.

5. Put the mixture into the refrigerator to let cool. As it cools gently stir and help the exfoliants to suspend in the oils.

6. After about 45 minutes, pour into your molds and leave to cool. If you want to speed up the process, you can put them in your freezer.

7. If you make a mistake, you can just remelt and start again.

Ta-da! Your little pieces of body butter exfoliant joy are ready to use. Gently rub them over your skin as you would soap in the bath or shower. They will exfoliate while at the same time being incredibly moisturizing and they are so much fun to use!

#15 Simple Moisturizing Body Butter

This is probably the simplest body butter recipe out there, but keep in mind because it uses baby lotion it is likely to contain chemicals and preservatives.

Ingredients:

- 16 ounces baby lotion
- 8 ounces solid coconut oil
- 8 ounces Vitamin E cream

Instructions:

1. Mix together with your mixer until it resembles icing.
2. Place in glass jars and seal.

#16 Jojoba and Shea Butter Whipped Body Butter

Ingredients

- ½ cup Jojoba oil
- ½ cup Shea butter
- ½ cup coconut oil
- 10-20 drops lavender essential oil

Directions

1. Place Shea butter, coconut oil and Jojoba oil in a glass bowl or measuring cup inside a saucepan. The saucepan should have enough water in it that the water touches the bottom of your glass double boiler, but doesn't spill out.
2. Over medium heat, whisk the oils together until they are melted and combined.
3. The mixture will go from white to semi-clear when ready.
4. Refrigerate melted oils for an hour or until white and solid.
5. With a stand mixer or hand mixer, beat the oils until they are fluffy like whipped cream. Add essential oils and beat to incorporate.
6. Fill your desired container with the whipped body butter and refrigerate another hour.

This body butter will keep about 6 months at room temperature. It may soften in warm weather because of the coconut oil. If this happens it can be stored in the refrigerator.

It is especially when you use it after a scrub.

#17 Jojoba and Lavender Relaxing Body Butter

This is a lovely smelling body butter and
it will help to relax your muscles.

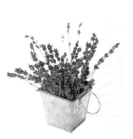

Ingredients:

- ½ cup Jojoba oil
- ½ cup Shea butter
- ½ cup coconut oil
- 10-20 drops lavender essential oil

Instructions:

1. Place the Shea butter, Jojoba oil and coconut oil in a double boiler.
2. Over medium heat, mix the oils together until they are melted and blended.
3. Your mixture will turn from white to semi-clear when ready.
4. Refrigerate your melted oils for about an hour or until they turn white and solid.
5. With your mixer, beat the oils until they are fluffy and resemble whipped cream.
6. Add your essential oils and beat to mix them in.
7. Fill your glass jars and seal.

8. Refrigerate another hour.

The Jojoba and lavender body butter will last about 6 months at room temperature. It can become too soft in warm weather because of the coconut oil and you can refrigerate if you like.

#18 Jojoba and Peppermint Refreshing Body Butter

This is a lovely smelling body butter and it will help leave you feeling refreshed.

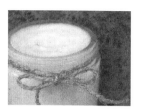

Ingredients:

- ½ cup Jojoba oil
- ½ cup Shea butter
- ½ cup coconut oil
- 10-20 drops peppermint essential oil

Instructions:

1. Place the Shea butter, Jojoba oil and coconut oil in a double boiler.
2. Over medium heat, mix the oils together until they are melted and blended.
3. Your mixture will turn from white to semi-clear when ready.
4. Refrigerate your melted oils for about an hour or until they turn white and solid.
5. With your mixer beat the oils until they are fluffy and resemble whipped cream.
6. Add your essential oils and beat to mix them in.
7. Fill your glass jars and seal.

8. Refrigerate another hour.

The Jojoba and peppermint body butter will last about 6 months at room temperature. It can become too soft in warm weather because of the coconut oil and you can refrigerate if you like.

#19 Lavender Body Butter

This simple, relaxing, and rejuvenating lavender body butter is

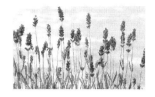 soothing to the skin and great for use on a

sunburn.

Ingredients:

- 8 tablespoons coconut oil
- 3 tablespoons olive oil
- 4 tablespoons beeswax
- 2 teaspoons honey
- 6 tablespoons Aloe Vera gel
- 4 teaspoons lanolin
- 25 drops lavender essential oil
- 2 Vitamin E capsules

Directions:

1. In double boiler over medium heat, add the oils, beeswax and honey.
2. In a separate double boiler over medium heat, add aloe.
3. Once melted, mix into beeswax mixture and stir.
4. Add lanolin and stir.
5. Once mixture has melted, turn heat to low.
6. Stir in Vitamin E and essential oil.

7. Whip until smooth.

8. Pour into small glass jars and let cool before covering.

#20 Rosemary Mint Whipped Shea Body Butter

This luxuriously whipped moisturizing creation instantly penetrates your skin and it will provide long-lasting protection and moisture. Kukui Nut Oil is highly penetrable and soothing.

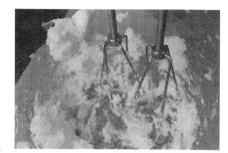

It can help soothe chapped skin as it contains high levels of the essential fatty acids linolenic acid and alpha-linolenic, which makes is perfect for dry skin, eczema, psoriasis and sensitive skin.

Ingredients:

- 4 ounces cocoa butter
- 7 ounces Shea butter
- 7 ounces Kukui nut oil
- 50 drops spearmint essential oil
- 25 drops rosemary essential oil

Directions:

1. In a double boiler measure out your cocoa butter.
2. Add in your Shea butter. Shea butter is soft, so you can easily scoop it out of the jar.

3. Drizzle in the Kukui nut oil.

4. Place the over medium heat and allow the butters and oil melt.

5. Allow the melted mixture to cool at room temp for about 15 minutes.

6. Transfer to your freezer for 20-30 minutes.

7. Blend the mixture with a whisk attachment for about 5 minutes. Place back into the freezer for about 20 minutes until it is super cold.

8. It should be starting to turn a creamy color. Keep whisking.

9. Scrape down the bowl sides as needed.

10. Add your essential oils.

11. Use your body butter within 60 days. Store in a cool and dark place.

#21 Mango Citrus Body Butter

Ingredients:

- 1 ounce beeswax wax
- 2 ounces cocoa butter
- 2 ounces Shea butter
- 2 ounces mango butter
- 4 teaspoon almond oil
- 2 teaspoon vitamin E
- 55 drops citrus essential oils -30 lime, 10 sweet orange, 15 lemon

Instructions:

1. Melt the beeswax, mango butter and cocoa butter in a double boiler on low-medium heat.
2. Leave the mixture over a gentle heat for 20 minutes to prevent the butter from going grainy when it cools.
3. Add your almond oil and Vitamin E
4. Heat for a few more minutes until it is completely liquid.
5. Remove from the heat
6. Add your essential oils while stirring thoroughly
7. Pour into jars and leave to set.

#22 Coconut Rose Body Butter

Ingredients:

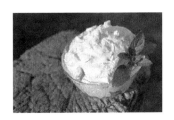

- 60 grams refined Coconut oil
- 1 ounce Jojoba oil
- 1 teaspoon Alkanet infused oil
- ½ ounce cornstarch
- 20 drops Rose essential oil

Instructions:

1. Place the coconut oil, Jojoba oil; Alkanet infused oil and cornstarch in our double boiler.
2. Heat the mixture until the coconut oil is melted.
3. Whisk to mix all ingredients.
4. Let cool to room temp.
5. Once mixture is cooled to room temp, add your essential oil.
6. Whisk until fluffy. It will resemble frosting.
7. Put into a glass jar and seal.
8. Store below 70 degrees for best results.
9. Use within 3 months.

#23 Almond Body Butter

Ingredients:

- 2 cup organic raw solid Shea butter
- 1 cup solid coconut oil
- 1 cup liquid almond oil

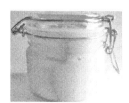

Instructions:

1. Melt the Shea butter and coconut oil in the top of your double boiler.
2. Remove from heat and let cool for 30-50 minutes.
3. Stir in the almond oil and essential oils.
4. Place the oil mixture in the freezer to chill.
5. Wait until your oils start to partially solidify.
6. Then whip until you achieve a butter-like consistency.
7. Place in clean glass jar and seal
8. Enjoy! A little will go a long way.

Tips:

- If you are allergic to any of the oils you can substitute as you like. Just keep the ratio the same and replace with the same type. For example, solid oil with solid oil. This will ensure that you can whip it and get the correct consistency.

- Chilling properly is key to your success. If you do not properly chill it will whip, but it won't stay whipped.
- This recipe needs to be stored in a cool place, but it does not have to be refrigerated. It should last at least a couple of months, even longer.
- This body butter is a little oily, but it absorbs quickly and leaves your skin very soft and supple.

- You can adjust your essential oils to what makes you happy as far as fragrance strength.

#24 Super Glowy Jasmine Body Butter

Ingredients:

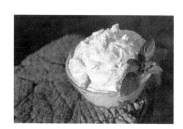

- 4 cups Extra Virgin, Raw & Organic Coconut Oil
- 14 ounces Shea Butter
- 2 drops Tea Tree Oil
- 20 drops of lemon, jasmine and spearmint essential oils

Instructions:

1. Add Coconut oil and Shea butter to your double-boiler and on medium heat let liquefy.
2. Remove from the heat.
3. Add your tea tree oil and jasmine essential oils and blend for 1 minute.
4. Allow to cool and solidify. If want to speed up this process you can put the bowl in the refrigerator.
5. Once solid, whip until smooth and fluffy.
6. Place in your glass jars and seal.

Tips:

Two other excellent essential oil blends are Sweet orange and lemon, peppermint, lavender, and basil. Don't be afraid to experiment with the essential oils. You may already have your own favorite combination.

#25 Whipped Argan & Mango Body Butter

This recipe is a little more complex than some others and a 'heads up' because it does contain some ingredients that you might not normally have in your home, but it's a very good recipe and worth taking the time to try. It's one that many spas like to use.

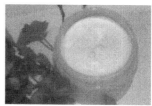

Ingredients:

Part 1 Ingredients

- 1 ½ ounces Ritamulse emulsifying wax
- ½ ounce cetyl alcohol
- 1 ounce mango butter
- ½ ounce Argan oil
- 2 ounces apricot kernel oil
- 1 ounce cocoa butter
- ¼ ounce glycerin
- 1 ounce Aloe Vera extract
- 1 teaspoon allantoin
- 2 teaspoon dimethicone

Part 2 Ingredients

- 10 ounces boiling water

Part 3 Ingredients

- 1 teaspoon phytokeratin
- 1 teaspoon geogard preservative
- 2 teaspoons dry flo

Instructions:

1. In a large mixing bowl, weigh out all the ingredients of Part #1.
2. Just before you start to measure, get your water boiling so that it is ready once you are done measuring.
3. Once your water has boiled, add Part #2 to Part #1.
4. Then mix well.
5. Put the mixture into your double boiler on medium heat until all the solids are melted and there are no chunks remaining.
6. Whisk fairly vigorously for a couple of minutes, and you will begin to see the texture change to a creamy, pudding-like consistency.
7. Take the butter's temperature. You want to make sure it is less than 113 degrees Fahrenheit or 45 degrees Celsius.
8. Once it has cooled to below 113 Fahrenheit, pop it back on the scale and weigh out the ingredients of Part #3 directly into the cream.

9. If the temperature of the butter is higher than what is recommended it could lead to damage of the vitamins, proteins, and preservatives that you add here.

10. Whisk very gently so as to avoid a cloud of powder flying up in your face.

11. Mix well until there are no visible clumps.

12. Get your electric hand mixer out, and whip your butter. This creates tiny air bubbles that lend to a lighter skin feel to the cream and also increase the volume. Continue to whip it until you get the desired consistency. Remember the more you whip it the fluffier it is going to be, so the more jars you are going to need.

13. Put into glass jars and seal.

Tip:

One of the easiest ways to get fluffy cream into a jar is by piping it in. If you don't have a commercial piper just put the lotion into a Ziploc bag and snip the corner. Then pipe the lotion into the bottle like you would put icing on a cake.

This recipe leaves your skin silky soft and your skin will feel so luxurious after. It also protects and heals dry, chapped skin without feeling oily.

#26 Cinnamon Body Butter for Cellulite

Cinnamon has some rather great qualities that include anti-fungal, antibacterial and antimicrobial qualities. It has astringent qualities that similar to Witch Hazel and it is rich in minerals like Iron, calcium and magnesium that are known to keep your skin healthy.

Wait - there's more! Cinnamon helps local blood circulation and therefore it can spread the distribution of cellulite, which is why it is the perfect addition in a body butter. It helps to remove blood impurities, reduce inflammation and heal cellulite.

Ingredients:

- 1/3 ounce coconut oil
- 2 ounces cocoa butter
- 2 ounces Shea butter
- 40 drops of cinnamon oil
- Cinnamon Stick

Instructions:

1. On your stove in your double boiler, on medium heat, warm the cocoa butter and Shea Butter until it becomes liquid.
2. Slowly stir in the coconut oil for about a minute.
3. Turn off the heat.
4. Let the mixture cool for 15 to 20 minutes. Don't let it set too fast.
5. As soon as it is cool, add the cinnamon oil.
6. Whip the mixture until it becomes light and fluffy.
7. Break pieces of the cinnamon stick into the mixture.
8. Place it into glass jars and seal, so that it keeps its consistency.

#27 Chocolate Body Butter Recipe

This is great all year round, but since it is edible, it is especially a great one to make at Valentine's Day because it is edible. Now you and your lover can both enjoy this great recipe.

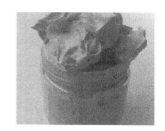

Once prepared, you can keep this recipe at room temperature and use it where ever and whenever your heart desires.

Ingredients:

- 1 ¼ cup coconut oil, melted
- ¾ cup clear agave nectar
- 1 tablespoon vanilla powder
- ½ cup cacao powder – you can add slightly more if you want a thicker mix

Instructions:

1. Place all the ingredients into a food processor
2. Blend until all the ingredients are well mixed/blended.
3. Pour into small glass jars and let the mixture set up in the fridge.
4. You can keep it at room temperature in a cool place.

Add-Ons Options:

- ½ teaspoon cistanche (promote sexual prowess)
- 2 teaspoon maca (balances hormones and strengthens libido)
- 2 to 4 drops rose essential oil
- 1 teaspoon powdered lavender flowers

#28 Coffee Butter Foot Cream

Rub this cream into your tired feet for an indulgent treat. The beeswax makes it a nice thick consistency and the Peppermint essential oil gives the feet a pick-me-up. Adding the dark rich chocolate fragrance oil enhances the coffee butter's natural aroma

Ingredients:

- 0.7 ounces white beeswax
- 3.5 ounces coffee butter
- 2 ounces sunflower oil
- 1 ounce stearic acid
- 1 ounce emulsifying wax
- 16 ounces distilled water
- 5 ml dark, rich chocolate fragrance oil
- 20 drops Peppermint
- 0.2 ounces Optiphen

Instructions:

1. In a double boiler, combine and melt the emulsifying wax, stearic Acid, beeswax, sunflower oil and coffee butter.

2. In a separate heat-safe container, heat the distilled water. Aim for 150-155 degrees in order to keep the Beeswax in the oil mixture melted as it emulsifies.

3. Check the temperature of the oil mixture. Once the temperature is reached, add the oils to the water and stick 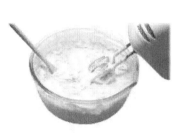 blend continuously for about 3 to 4 minutes.

4. The preservative Optiphen can't be added to a temperature that is higher than 176 degrees or it will be useless. Once you are sure that the temperature is good you can add the Optiphen, dark rich chocolate fragrance oil and peppermint essential oil.

5. Stick blend for another minute or so.

6. Let cool a bit

7. While it is still warm, pour it into your glass jars.

8. Allow the glass jars to sit for 24 hours and then seal. This will give it lots of time to cool so there's no condensation on the inside.

9. Enjoy!

#29 Dreamy Homemade Lemon Cream Body Butter Recipe

This body butter is so rich and luxurious that you are going to love it. It's great for dry or scaly skin and it will do a great job of keeping your skin hydrated and soft all year round.

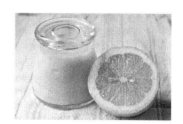

Ingredients:

- 12 Tablespoons coconut oil
- ½ cup cacao butter
- 2 Tablespoon Vitamin E oil
- 1 Teaspoon lemon essential oil

Instructions:

1. Place the coconut oil and cacao butter in a saucepan.
2. On low heat, warm until it just melts.
3. Remove from the heat.
4. Add the Vitamin E oil and essential oil.
5. Cool until the mixture solidifies. This will take a few hours.
6. Pour into glass jars and seal. It will last a couple of months.

This is one of the most delightful body butters you'll find. Not only is it not greasy, it smells fabulous!

#30 Decadent Whipped Body Butter

Ingredients:

- 2 cups of cocoa butter
- 1 cup coconut oil
- 1 cup of Jojoba oil or almond oil

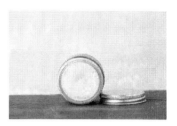

Instructions:

1. Use a double boiler on medium heat to gently but completely melt your cocoa butter and coconut oil.
2. Stir in Jojoba or almond oil.
3. Allow to chill in the refrigerator until the oil mixture begins to firm. Do not let it turn solid. This will take at least several hours.
4. Use your mixer and whip the semi-solid mixture until white peaks form.
5. Put into glass jars and allow to chill for an hour in the fridge.
6. Seal your glass jars.

This homemade lotion will stay whipped in moderate temperatures. If your home is on the warm side, it is best to store it in the refrigerator. If your whipped butter melts back to oil, just re-chill it and whip it again.

This whipped body butter leaves a thin layer of oil for your body to drink up.

#31 Pretty in Pink Body Butter

Ingredients:

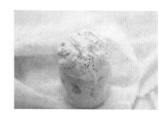

- 2 cup Coconut Oil
- 3 cups vegetable shortening
- 4 drops pink food dye
- 10-20 drops of your favorite essential oils

Instructions:

1. In a large bowl, place the coconut oil, vegetable shortening and 2 drops of food dye.
2. Use your mixer and combine all the ingredients until they become a pink whip.
3. Add 2 more drops of food coloring and your favorite essential oils.
4. Take your rubber spatula and whip the butter until the essential oils and dye have been incorporated.
5. Place in glass jars and seal.

#32 Homemade Coconut Vanilla Body Butter

Ingredients:

12 Tablespoons coconut oil

1/2 cup cacao butter

2 Tablespoon Vitamin E oil

20-30 drops of vanilla essential oil

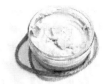

Instructions:

1. Place the coconut oil and cacao butter in a saucepan. Over low heat until it melts
2. Remove from the heat.
3. Add your Vitamin E oil and vanilla essential oil.
4. At room temperature cool until the mixture solidifies, which will take at least a couple of hours.
5. Put in glass jars and seal.

#33 Honey and Lemon Body Butter

This is a great moisturizer as it helps your skin to retain water, leaving it smooth and supple. It is also great for reducing fine lines and wrinkles. The smell of citrus oils makes this butter smell decadent.

Instructions:

- 4 tablespoons of beeswax
- 1 cup of grapeseed oil
- 2 capsules of vitamin e oil
- 3-5 tablespoons distilled water
- 20 drops of citrus essential oils

Instructions:

1. In a double boiler, combine the grapeseed oil, beeswax and Vitamin E and then heat until the beeswax just melts.
2. Using your mixer and beat the oils on high while you add the distilled water a little bit at a time. The mixture will turn from oily to milky.
3. You control the body butter thickness by how much water you add, but the recommended amount is 3 to 5 tablespoons.

4. Once the desired consistency is achieved, add your citrus essential oil.

5. Turn off the mixer and let the lotion sit for 15-20 minutes, then place into glass jars and seal.

#34 Eczema Fighting Body Butter

Ingredients:

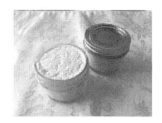

- 4 ounces of Shea butter
- 1 ounce avocado oil
- 3 Vitamin E capsules

Instructions:

1. Put the Shea butter and avocado oil in a double boiler over medium heat and let melt.
2. When they were completely melted and mixed take them off the heat and added the Vitamin E.
3. Let it cool to room temperature.
4. Whip it up into a meringue like consistency.
5. Put into glass jars, seal and store in refrigerator.
6. It almost immediately melts when it hits your skin. Apply 2 to 3 times a day.

#35 Christmas Mango and Mint Body Butter

Ingredients:

- 1cup Shea butter
- 1 cup mango butter
- 1 cup coconut oil
- 1 cup light almond oil
- Use 20-30 drops of spearmint essential oil
- 3 to 4 drops green or red food dye

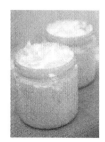

Instructions:

1. In a double combine all the ingredients except essential oils and food dye.
2. On medium heat stir constantly until all the ingredients are melted.
3. Add your food dye and mix in thoroughly
4. Remove from heat and let it slightly cool.
5. Move to your refrigerator and let cool for another hour or until starting to harden but still somewhat soft.
6. Use your mixer and whip until fluffy.
7. Return to refrigerator for 15 to 20 minutes to set.
8. Put into a glass jar and seal.

9. If your home stays above 75 degrees, store in the refrigerator so that it stays whipped.

#36 Coconut & Plum Whipped Body Butter

Ingredients:

- 4 ounces organic virgin coconut cream oil
- 4 ounces ultra refined cocoa butter
- 2 ounces plum kernel oil
- 1 ounce carnauba wax
- 3 teaspoons plum Jojoba wax beads

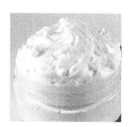

Instructions:

1. In a double boiler over medium-high heat, combine the cocoa butter, virgin coconut oil, and waxes.
2. It is important to heat these ingredients gently until they have melted completely.
3. Add the Plum Kernel Oil.
4. Remove the mixture from the heat.
5. Place the double boiler into a pot of ice water, and continuously and vigorously whip until thickened. This can take several minutes, even with an electric mixer. It can help to move the boiler in/out of the ice bath to control the thickness of the mixture.
6. Make sure the mixture doesn't stick to the sides of the boiler.

7. When the mixture has thickened to where it has become thick and fluffy like frosting you can place into your glass jars.

8. Allow the mixture to set in the containers completely before handling. This can take several hours. Then seal.

#37 Orange & Coconut Whipped Body Butter

Ingredients:

- 1 cup coconut oil
- 2 tablespoons Shea butter
- 4 drops sweet almond oil
- 50 drops orange essential oil

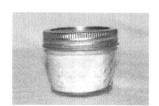

Instructions:

1. Place the coconut oil, Shea butter, and sweet almond oil in a medium-sized bowl.
2. Use your mixer to beat the ingredients for a few minutes to combine them.
3. Add the essential oil and continue to mix for 6 to 8 minutes or until the mixture is fluffy. Use a rubber spatula to scrape down the sides of the bowl when necessary.
4. Put into glass jars and seal. If you live in a warm climate refrigerate so your body butter doesn't melt.

#38 Eucalyptus Mint Whipped Body Butter

Ingredients:

- 1 cup coconut oil
- 12 tablespoons Shea butter
- 12 tablespoons cocoa butter
- 2 tablespoon carrier oil
- 3 teaspoons castor oil
- 20 drops eucalyptus essential oil
- 6 drops peppermint essential oil

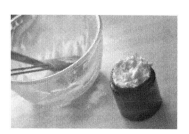

Instructions:

1. In a small double boiler over low-medium heat, warm the coconut oil, Shea butter, and cocoa butter until softened. Transfer to a medium bowl.
2. Add in the castor oil, carrier oil, eucalyptus essential oil, and the peppermint essential oil.
3. Stir together.
4. Place the bowl in the refrigerator until the oils are soft and thick. This usually takes several hours.
5. When the mixture is firm but not hard, remove from the refrigerator and whip with your mixer until it is soft and fluffy. Transfer to glass jars and seal.

#39 Wild Orange Body Butter Recipe

Ingredients:

- 2 cups shaved cocoa butter
- 1 to 2 tablespoons of almond oil
- 10 drops of Vitamin E oil
- 10 drops of Wild Orange essential oil

Instructions:

1. Soften the cocoa butter in your double boiler over medium heat.
2. Whip up the cocoa butter with your mixer and slowly add your almond oil.
3. Add in the Vitamin E oil and your essential oils and stir together until well mixed.
4. Pour into glass jars and seal. It should last approx. 3 months.

#40 Honey Kissed Massage Body Butter

Ingredients:

1 ½ cups cocoa butter

1 ½ cups Shea butter

4 tablespoons Apricot Kernel oil

2 capsules Vitamin E oil

2 tablespoons honey powder

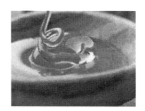

Instructions:

1. Put about an inch of water in the bottom of a medium-sized pot and heat to a low simmer.

2. Place the cocoa and Shea butter in a large heat-proof glass measuring cup.

3. Place the measuring cup in the water and warm it slowly over a low heat until the butters melt.

4. Cook at a low heat for approx. 20 minutes. Do not let it boil.

5. Remove from the heat and add the rest of the ingredients.

6. Use a metal spoon to combine the ingredients, stirring continuously.

7. Use a mixer to whip the butter continually for several minutes in the same manner that you would with frosting. It will begin to look like whipped cream.

8. Spoon into glass jars. Reduce air bubbles by sharply tapping on the counter occasionally as you fill. Seal and store.

#41 Aromatherapy Lavender & Rose Flower Body Butter

Ingredients:

- ½ cup cocoa butter
- 2 cups Shea butter
- 4 tablespoons Sweet Almond oil
- 2 tablespoon Jojoba oil
- 2 tablespoon Rosehip oil
- 2 capsules Vitamin E
- 2 teaspoon Corn Starch
- 40 drops Lavender essential oil
- 10 drops Frankincense essential oil
- 4 drops Palmarosa essential oil
- 4 drops Rose Geranium essential oil

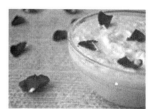

Instructions:

1. Put about an inch of water in the bottom of a medium-sized pot and heat to a low simmer.
2. Place the cocoa and Shea butter in a large heat-proof glass measuring cup.
3. Place the measuring cup in the water and warm it slowly over a low heat until the butters melt.

4. Cook at a low heat for approx. 20 minutes. Do not let it boil.

5. Remove from the heat and add the rest of the ingredients.

6. Use a metal spoon to combine the ingredients, stirring continuously.

7. Use a mixer to whip the butter continually for several minutes in the same manner that you would with frosting. It will begin to look like whipped cream.

8. Spoon into glass jars. Reduce air bubbles by sharply tapping on the counter occasionally as you fill. Seal and store.

#42 Aromatherapy Lavender Spice Body Butter

Ingredients:

- ½ cup cocoa butter
- 2 cups Shea butter
- 4 tablespoons Sweet Almond oil
- 2 tablespoon Jojoba oil
- 2 tablespoon Rosehip oil
- 2 capsules Vitamin E
- 2 teaspoon Corn Starch
- 40 drops Lavender essential oil
- 8 drops Patchouli essential oil
- 8 drops Sandalwood essential oil
- 4 drops Cedarwood essential oil

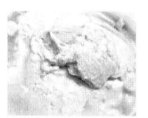

Instructions:

1. Put about an inch of water in the bottom of a medium-sized pot and heat to a low simmer.
2. Place the cocoa and Shea butter in a large heat-proof glass measuring cup.
3. Place the measuring cup in the water and warm it slowly over a low heat until the butters melt.
4. Cook at a low heat for approx. 20 minutes. Do not let it boil.

5. Remove from the heat and add the rest of the ingredients.

6. Use a metal spoon to combine the ingredients, stirring continuously.

7. Use a mixer to whip the butter continually for several minutes in the same manner that you would with frosting. It will begin to look like whipped cream.

8. Spoon into glass jars. Reduce air bubbles by sharply tapping on the counter occasionally as you fill. Seal and store.

#43 Varicose Vein Attacking Body Butter

Ingredients:

- 1 cup Shea butter
- ½ cup coconut oil
- ½ cup Jojoba oil
- 2 capsules Vitamin E
- 10 drops of cypress essential oil
- 10 drops of lemon essential oil
- 5 drops of fennel essential oil
- 5 drops helichrysum essential oil

Instructions:

1. Heat the Shea butter and coconut oil in a double boiler on medium low.
2. Stir until the oils melt, just a few minutes.
3. Remove from heat.
4. Add the Jojoba oil, Vitamin E capsules, and essential oils.
5. Refrigerate for about an hour or until chilled. It will be off-white, almost solid.
6. Use your mixer to beat until you have soft white peaks like with

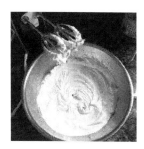

whip cream.

7. Place in glass jars and seal.

Massage this towards your heart to improve your blood flow. Start at your ankles and work up your legs, start at your wrists and work up towards your shoulders, etc.

Your body butter should last about 6 months. You can store it at room temperature. During the hot weather, store in the refrigerator.

#44 Tangerine Whipped Body Butter

Ingredients:

1 cup Shea butter

½ cup organic coconut oil

½ cup sweet almond oil

20 drops tangerine essential oil

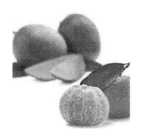

Instructions:

1. Combine all the ingredients in a medium size bowl.
2. Using your mixer, whip ingredients until peaks form like whip cream. The texture will be a little thicker than whipped cream.
3. Put into glass jars and seal.

Your body butter should last about 6 months. You can store it at room temperature. During the hot weather, store in the refrigerator.

#45 Mountain Rose Herb Body Butter

Ingredients:

- 6 ounces Shea butter
- 4 ounces mango butter
- 2 ounces coconut oil
- 6 ounces grapeseed oil
- 1 ounce beeswax4 ounces distilled water or hydrosol
- 4 ounces Aloe Vera gel
- 100 drops of sweet orange with 100 drops of patchouli, 30 drops of lavender essential oils.

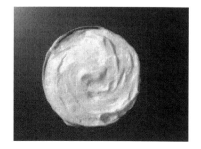

Instructions:

1. Combine all your butters, oils and wax into your double boiler and place on medium heat until melted, while occasionally stirring.
2. When the oils, butters, and wax have melted, pour into your blender; let it come to room temperature.
3. Measure out the distilled water and Aloe Vera gel and let it come to room temperature.
4. When the butter/oil/wax mixture has cooled enough it will be thick and opaque.

5. Only then, turn on the blender and slowly add the water/Aloe Vera gel. The color will lighten significantly and the mixture will be one homogenous consistency.

6. If necessary, scrape down the sides and continue blending.

7. When the body butter is fully blended, add your essential oils.

8. When the body butter is exactly how you want it, pour it into your jars, and seal.

9. As it cools the body butter will firm up. If you want, you can keep your body butter at room temperature but if you refrigerate it, you'll increase its life expectancy.

Body butter can be messy to clean up after. Use paper towel to wipe as much as possible off everything and then try washing.

#46 Mint Chocolate Whipped Body Butter

Ingredients:

- 1 cup of organic cocoa butter
- 1 cup organic mango butter.
- 1 cup coconut oil
- 1 cup of Jojoba. Almond oil can also be used, but it will decrease shelf life because it is more vulnerable to oxidation.
- 2 to 4 teaspoons peppermint essential oil – this is personal
- 4 tablespoons pure cocoa or cacao powder.
- 4 teaspoons naturally derived Vitamin E

Instructions:

1. Prepare an ice bath by filling one of your large bowls with ice and fitting it into a smaller bowl inside. The inside bowl needs to hold a minimum of 5 cups of liquid.
2. Use a double boiler to melt the cocoa butter and mango butter over a low simmer.
3. Add coconut oil and melt until it is all liquid.
4. Remove the cocoa butter/coconut oil mixture from the heat.

5. Measure 2 tablespoons of cocoa powder into a small bowl and slowly add several tablespoons of Jojoba oil.
6. Mix thoroughly and then add it to the cocoa butter/coconut oil mixture along with the rest of the Jojoba oil.
7. Place mixture in chilled bowl and let cool for 10 minutes.
8. Remove the mixture from the ice bath and whip until the peaks are stiff peaks. If in a few minutes it isn't starting to thicken, return the bowl to the ice bath and whip there.
9. Place in glass jars and seal. Store away from the sun.

Tips:

- If you would like a "white chocolate" version that is not a bronzer, so you can substitute arrowroot powder or non-GMO cornstarch.
- This recipe contains no preservatives, but the oils and butters themselves have been selected because they are naturally antimicrobial. When quality oils are used, this body butter can stay fresh at room temp between 3 to 6 months without using Vitamin E. If you use Vitamin E it can stay fresh for up to a year.

#47 Whipped Peppermint Bark Body Butter

Ingredients:

- ½ cups cocoa butter
- ½ cups Shea butter
- ½ cups coconut oil
- 4 capsules Vitamin E
- ½ teaspoon peppermint extract

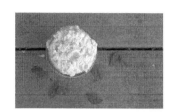

Instructions:

1. Measure the first four ingredients into a microwave-safe bowl. If you are using the kind of cocoa butter that comes in a jar, heat it in the microwave until it is soft enough to scoop out. It takes about two minutes.
2. Microwave all of the oils until they are melted, which takes about three minutes. If any small solid pieces remain, stir until they are completely melted and mixed in.
3. Stir in peppermint extract.
4. Place the bowl in the freezer and cool for 15 to 20 minutes, until about ¾ of the oil is solid but soft.
5. Transfer the oils to the bowl of a mixing bowl and whip until light and fluffy. Scrape the sides with a rubber spatula every couple of minutes.

6. Transfer to glass jars and seal.

7. Enjoy!

#48 Calming Orange Vanilla Whipped Body Butter

Ingredients:

- 1 ½ cups coconut oil
- 1 ½ cups Shea butter
- 2 tablespoons Jojoba oil
- 2 tablespoons Vitamin E oil
- 20 drops of lavender essential oil
- 40 drops of orange essential oil
- 2 teaspoons vanilla extract

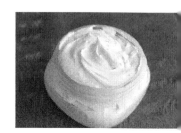

Instructions:

1. Put the coconut oil and Shea butter in the bowl, and then mix using your hand mixer.
2. Start on low speed until everything is incorporated.
3. Then turn the mixer up to high speed and whip the coconut oil and Shea butter until they're a light and fluffy whipped mixture.
4. Add in the Jojoba, Vitamin E, essential oils and vanilla.
5. Whip again with the mixer until just incorporated.
6. Place in glass jars, seal, and let cool in a dark place.

#49 Cranberry Body Butter Whip

Ingredients:

- ½ cup coconut oil
- 2 tablespoons Shea butter
- 2 tablespoons frozen cranberries
- 2 drops orange essential oil, optional

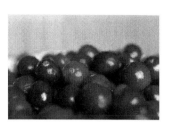

Instructions:

1. In a large bowl, add the coconut oil and Shea butter.
2. With your mixer, mix the ingredients for 5-8 minutes.
3. Add your cranberries to a small food processor and pulse until they become small pieces.
4. Add the cranberries to your coconut oil mixture.
5. Place the mixture in a fine mesh sieve and press it through with a spatula to a clean bowl. This will keep the pieces of cranberries out of the butter.
6. Add the essential oil and mix it with a spoon.
7. Transfer the mixture to small glass jars and seal. It will keep one week not refrigerated.

#50 Sugar Cookie Body Butter

Ingredients:

- 3.5 ounces cocoa butter
- 3.5 ounces Shea butter
- 3.5 ounces mango butter
- 1.6 ounces Argan oil
- 1.8 ounces fractionated coconut oil
- 4 capsules Vitamin E
- 1 ounce sugar cookies fragrance oil

Instructions:

1. Weigh out of your butters and the Argan and fractionated coconut oils.
2. In a double boiler over medium heat completely melt the butters and weighed out oils. Be careful not to get the oils too hot, or it could ruin them.
3. Once melted, remove them from your heat source and your Vitamin E capsules and sugar cookies fragrance.
4. Stir.
5. Pour the mixture into your mixing bowl and then place it in another bowl filled with ice. This helps to cool it faster. If you have no ice, you can cover and set it in the refrigerator to cool.

6. As it cools the mixture will get thicker.

7. Every 20 minutes or so, use your hand mixer to whip the butter for several minutes. After each mix, place the mixture back into the fridge or over the ice bowl for additional cooling and thickening purposes.

8. The mixture will start to get thicker every time you mix it and it will begin to look like whipped butter.

9. Once the butter has solidified all the way and is no longer runny, put it into your glass jars and seal.

#51 Strawberry Body Butter

Ingredients:

- 4 ounces Shea butter
- 3 teaspoons Jojoba oil
- 3 teaspoons apricot oil
- 2 ounces coconut oil
- ½ teaspoon of strawberry food flavoring
- A couple of drops of red food coloring

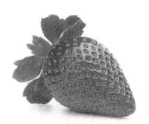

Instructions:

1. Mix all your ingredients together
2. Add your flavoring to the mixture and mix again.
3. Once mixed store it in a glass jar and apply generously to your skin.

#51 Avocado Body Butter

This avocado body butter will do more than soothe your skin. It has natural sun blocking properties, provides joint pain relief, and has anti inflammatory qualities.

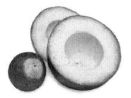

It's great for scars and it will protect you from environmental pollutants. The avocado oils is high in sterolin, Vitamins A, D, and E, with anti inflammatory and antibacterial qualities.

Ingredients:

- 32 ounces raw organic Shea butter
- 8 ounces raw organic cocoa butter
- ½ cup avocado oil
- 4 tablespoons vegetable glycerin

Instructions:

1. In your food processor, add the Shea butter.
2. Pulse it a couple of times to break it down.
3. Add in the vegetable glycerin and avocado oil.
4. Add the cocoa butter to a glass bowl and set in to a pot of hot water, but don't let the cocoa butter temperature go above 118 degrees in order for this to be a raw lotion.
5. Remove it from heat once things are well melted.
6. Continue stirring around. The heat will melt any little remaining chunks.
7. Now drizzle the cocoa butter into the food processor.
8. Mix until well incorporated into the mixture.
9. Put the lotion into glass jars and seal.

This can be a bit oily, but don't worry because eventually it will absorb into your skin. It's really thin in texture unlike most of the other recipes. That's the way it is supposed to be. As it cools, it will get somewhat firmer. This body butter keeps for months at room temperature.

#52 Lavender and Lace Body Butter

Ingredients:

- ½ cup coconut oil
- ½ cup Shea Butter
- ½ cup cocoa Butter
- 6 tablespoons Kukui Oil
- 2 capsules Vitamin E
- 2 teaspoons cornstarch
- 45-55 drops of Lavender essential oil

Instructions:

1. Microwave a large bowl of water until boiling.
2. Place the coconut oil, Shea butter and cocoa butter in a smaller glass bowl.
3. Set this bowl inside the hot water bath.
4. Stir with a metal spoon until it is completely melted and blended together.
5. You may need to reheat you water in the microwave to completely melt the butters.
6. Add the Kukui oil, Vitamin E and lavender oil.
7. Stir well.
8. Add the cornstarch and mix thoroughly.

9. Remove from the hot water bath and allow to cool for a few minutes.

10. Set the bowl of butters in an ice water bath. Use the same large bowl filled with ice and water.

11. With a hand mixer, whip up your body butter to a light as air consistency just like whipped cream. The more you whip the lighter and fluffier it is going to become.

12. Spoon into glass jars and seal.

Use after a shower by applying to damp skin to seal in moisture. You will love how your skin feels.

Main Ingredients Explained

A solid butter or carrier oil should be the main ingredient in all of your whipped body butter recipes. Shea butter has the correct texture to be used on its own, but other ingredients will need you to tweak them a little to get the best consistency.

Your butter should be firm enough to set up solid, but it needs to be soft enough to yield when you scoop it. Don't be afraid to experiment.

Shea Butter

Shea butter is derived from the nut of the African Shea tree. In the world of moisturizers it's become a bit of a rock star. It can

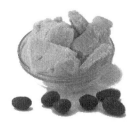 reduce the appearance of fine lines and wrinkles, and stretch marks, as well as soothe sunburn, and ease psoriasis and eczema.

It also contains beneficial fatty acids and has antioxidant and anti-inflammatory properties. And all of this without a greasy residue or a strong scent.

Mango

Mangos are a great source of fiber, Vitamin A, Vitamin C, and potassium. This tasty tropical fruit can do amazing things on your skin. Mango body butter is packed with antioxidants and, it can clear your pores.

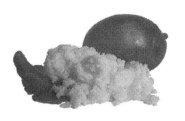

Coconut Oil

Many health experts report coconut oil to be the most beneficial of all the oils out there. It has been used for centuries to treat a wide range of ailments.

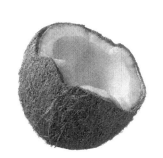

Studies show that it has anti inflammatory, antibacterial and antiviral properties, that it can help with tissue repair, increase your metabolism and so much more. It's also an excellent moisturizer and wrinkle-fighter.

Lavender

When lavender is added to body butter you get to enjoy the aromatherapeutic properties. Lavender is recognized for being a

stress and anxiety reliever, so the
next time you need a little
relaxation in your world, reach for
lavender body butter and enjoy
some top notch moisturizing too.

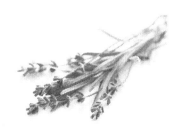

Cocoa

Cocoa butter is the fat from the cocoa bean. It is one of those
moisturizers that for centuries has been used around the world.

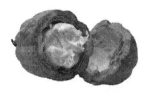

It has strong emollient properties,
stimulates collagen and elastin
production, reduces the appearance
of stretch marks and scars and
relieves eczema flare-ups. It also smells so good!

Kokum or Illipe Butters

These butters have a really hard
texture so you can use them by
themselves to create whipped butters.

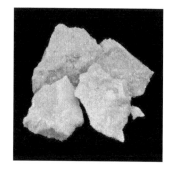

They will produce a slightly firmer
texture than you might want. To

soften you can add softer butters, or just a tiny amount of your carrier oil.

Almond

Almond oil is rich in Vitamin E, magnesium, calcium and fatty acids, which soothe eczema, irritation and itchiness.

For thousands of years, it has been used in Ayurvedic skin treatments. Almond oil has a light but calming scent that subtly relaxes your mind while doing magic for your skin.

Mandarin

Yes mandarin has a wonderful sweet smell of oranges, but it also has antiseptic properties and it promotes cell and tissue growth. It is known for its relaxing qualities and even for its role as a sedative. As far as body butter goes, it is an excellent moisturizer, wrinkle fighter and it will revive dull skin.

Olive Oil

You don't just cook with olive oil. It has terrific moisturizing qualities for extremely dry and sensitive skin. It may also fight cancer and sun damage. Many apply olive oil straight from the bottle onto their face and body, but olive body butter is a much nicer.

Hemp Oil

Hemp seed oil often gets a bad rap because of its connection to marijuana, but it is quickly becoming recognized as a versatile skin healer.

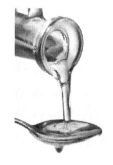

Hemp seed oil is unique because it has nearly 80% high fatty acid content along with a complete lineup of amino acids, which is rare. It is a natural antioxidant and an anti inflammatory agent. In fact, the chemical makeup of hemp seed oil is very close to that of our skin, so it can be easily absorbed and it will not clog your pores.

Coffee Bean, Macadamia, Pistachio

These butters are really soft, so you can't use them alone in a whipped body butter, as they will create a firm enough texture. You will need to blend them with a large portion of hard butters or waxes.

Aloe Vera

Aloe Vera is indeed a miracle plant. The gel that is found

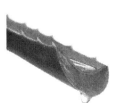

inside the Aloe Vera plant is an antioxidant often used to soothe sunburn, it aids with circulation, reduces skin inflammation, repairs skin tissue and it will cleanse the digestive system. Aloe Vera has a whopping 12 vitamins, 20 minerals, and 18 amino acids. It's also a good moisturizer.

Jojoba Oil

Jojoba oil is not really an oil, but rather a liquid wax that is derived from the seed of the jojoba plant. It has antibacterial, antiviral, and anti inflammatory properties. It will the moisture in your skin.

Tallow

Tallow closely resembles your own human cellular makeup. It
 contains 50 to 55% saturated fat just like our cell
membranes do and it is also very similar to your
skin's sebum, the waxy matter that lubricates and
waterproofs your skin.

Vitamin E

Vitamin E is a fat soluble antioxidant that is very important in
maintaining healthy skin. As an added bonus, it is also a natural
preservative that you can use in your homemade body butters.

Essential Oils

There are many essential oils that you can choose from. You
 can also make your own blend mixed up, to create
your own interesting fragrance.

 You should always use therapeutic grade essential
oils if you want to enjoy the therapeutic value and
not just the fragrance. Otherwise, you can use aromatherapy
grade essential oils.

- **Cheerful Citrus** -10 drops of each orange, bergamot and grapefruit, 3 drops of each rose ylang ylang and geranium.
- **Soothing Lavender**-14 drops each of orange and lavender, 4 drops of each ylang ylang and chamomile.

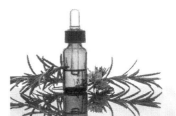

- **Sensual Rose** - 10 drops of each lavender, rose and palmarosa, 4 drops of each sage, clary and rose geranium.
- **Exotic Sandalwood** - 15 drops of sandalwood, 10 drops of patchouli, 10 drops of orange 2 drops each of ylang ylang, clove, ginger, and vetiver.

If you would like to reduce the strength of the scent you just need to decrease the number of essential oil drops you use.

Waxes

Waxes help to reinforce your whipped butters so that they are sturdier, firmer, and stickier. They will lend adhesion and body. Wax is really helpful in mixtures that use liquid oils or soft butters. Be careful that you don't add too much wax or you could land up with a product that is more similar to a balm than a butter and it can affect the pliability and texture of your mix.

Beeswax

Beeswax will add stickiness to the texture of your whipped body butter, so don't use too much. Add just enough to firm up your butter.

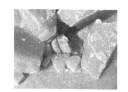

Candelilla Wax

You can use this vegetable-based wax to increase the firmness

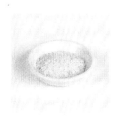

of your whipped body butter. It's much harder than either Jojoba or beeswax, so use sparingly in your recipes avoid adding having a sticky or brittle butter texture.

CO2 Extracts

These are ultra pure and very potent plant extracts that generally used because of their powerful herbal properties, but some CO2 extracts have an aroma that's desirable.

Attars

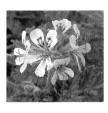 Attars are delicate floral extracts distilled in sandalwood. These rare aromatics are usually very expensive, and you should reserve their usage for your special whipped body butter recipes.

Fragrance Oils

Fragrance oils aren't natural, but rather they have been formulated for skin care products, which make them so easy to use, and you have tons of fragrances to choose from.

Additives

Additives are optional in your body butter recipes. They can help improve the slip, texture and longevity of your body butter. Cornstarch, Vitamin E, and silk powder are often used.

Cornstarch

Cornstarch will decrease the greasiness of your body butter, and it can make the texture of your formula more pleasant. You can add at a ratio of around 1 teaspoon per 1 - 2 ounces of main ingredients. Mix the cornstarch into a slurry with a little melted oil to avoid lumps.

Silk Powder

Silk Powder enhances the slip of body butter and you can add it at a rate of 1 - 5% of the total recipe.

Make it into a slurry prior to adding it to the melted ingredients. This will avoid lumps.

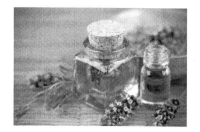

Antioxidants

Whipped body butters usually don't contain water or other fragile ingredients so you don't have to add a preservative. But you might like to include an antioxidant to help keep the essential oils and butters from oxidizing and going rancid prematurely.

Vitamin E is ideal for this purpose, and it will not affect the color or aroma of your body butter. Rosemary oil extract can also be used; however, it has a dark green color and herbal aroma that usually affects your finished product.

Basic Recipes for Whipped Body Butters

If you've used the recipes and are ready for something new, or you just want to understand the basics of body butter so you can

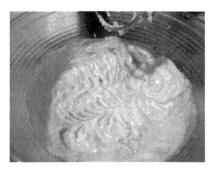

start experimenting, these basic recipes are a great place to start.

These recipes are for tiny batches so they are great for experimenting. Use a scale to measure all of your ingredients. As you are experimenting, take good notes, whether you are adding or subtracting additives, waxes, or aromatics.

Basic Whipped Shea Butter

Ingredients:

- 2 ounces Shea Butter
- 0.02 to 0.03 ounces (1-3%) Essential Oil **-or-**0.04 to 0.07 ounces (2-5%) Fragrance Oil

Basic Whipped Hard Butter

Ingredients:

- 1.4 ounces hard butter

- 0.01-0.03 ounces (1-3%) Essential Oil **-or-** 0.02 to 0.05 ounces (2-5%) Fragrance Oil
- 1 ounce liquid sweet almond as a carrier oil

Basic Whipped Medium-Soft Butter

Ingredients:

- 2 ounces Medium-Soft Butter like Mango
- 0.01-0.03 ounces (1-3%) Essential Oil **-or-** 0.02-1.5 ounces (2-5%) Fragrance Oil
- 0/05 ounces (5 - 10%) Wax

Basic Whipped Solid Oil

Ingredients:

- 1 ounce Solid Oil like coconut
- 15 grams Hard Butter (Cocoa, Kokum, etc.)
- 0.01-0.03 ounces (1-3%) Essential Oil **-or-** 0.02-0.05 ounces (2-5%) Fragrance Oil
- 0.10 – 0.21 ounces (10 - 20%) Wax

Basic Whipped Soft-Butter

Ingredients:

- 2 ounces Soft Butter like macadamia nut

- 0.01-0.03 ounces (1-3%) Essential Oil **-or-** 0.02-0.05 ounces (2-5%) Fragrance Oil
- 0.10 – 0.21 ounces (10 - 20%) Wax

Basic Directions for Whipped Body Butters

1. Melt butters, carrier oils and waxes together in a double boiler over medium heat.
2. When the mixture has melted completely you need to remove the boiler from heat.
3. Add any of the aromatics or additives.
4. Use your mixer to whip the mixture continuously as it starts cooling.
5. Continue whipping the butter until it cools and thickens. Remember to scrape the sides of the bowl as needed.
6. Do not quit whipping until the mixture becomes thick and fluffy. It should look like frosting.
7. Use your spatula to transfer the mixture to jars.
8. Let the butter cool, set, and harden completely before you use.

How to Buy Essential Oils

Poor quality oils, which could have been distilled from poor crops, handled improperly, be old, etc. are not therapeutic. Nor are oils that are adulterated, which have chemicals or other oils added to them.

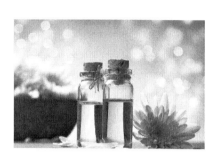

In addition essential oils that have chemicals associated with them can cause harmful side effects, and no therapeutic value. This is why when choosing oils for your body butter you want to look for therapeutic oils.

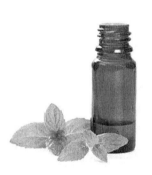

Do not make the mistake of assuming because you are applying the oils to your body and not taking them internally it doesn't matter – it does! Essential oils are absorbed through the skin and so you can enjoy many of the therapeutic qualities when you use quality oils.

Here are some tips to help you choose pure, high quality essential oils.

- Watch out for words such as fragrance oil, perfume oil, or nature identical oil. These words point towards something that isn't pure or a single essential oil. Many suppliers will label fragrance oils and perfume oils as 'aromatherapy 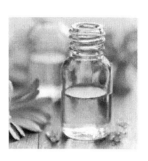 oils. You need to be aware of and watch out for these suppliers.

- Be cautious of suppliers that promote their essential oils as either being 'aromatherapy grade' or 'therapeutic 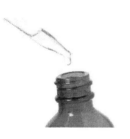 grade.' There is no governmental regulating body that certifies or grades essential oils as therapeutic or aromatherapy grade.

Not all companies will use these terms with the goal of deception, but some do. Don't base your buying decisions completely on the terminology that the vendor or supplier uses. Use all of the tips provided to ensure you feel comfortable with the supplier you are buying from.

- The term 'pure essential oil' is very overused in the aromatherapy industry as a whole. Pure essential oils can still be distilled from crops that are of poor or low quality.

They can have been sitting in inventory or on a store shelf for many years, making them less potent. They can be stored in a manner that results in damage to the oils. They can be mishandled by manufacturers so that leads to the accidental mixing during bottling.

What are we saying? Just don't be too impressed by a vendor that uses labels that say 'pure oils.' Dig deeper. Find out more about the vendor or supplier and make sure their reputation is one you can trust.

- Most vendors that sell high quality oils sell them in amounts that are 4 ounces or less and they sell them in dark colored glass, which helps to preserve them. Be cautious of suppliers or vendors that sell their oils at larger sizes or in clear glass or plastic containers.

- When you buy oils online, often larger sizes of essential oils are shipped in plastic containers to ensure breakage does not occur and it helps to lower the shipping costs. However, the essential oils can dissolve plastic bottles 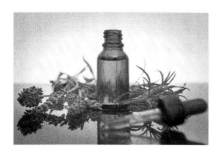 and the quality of the oil can rapidly deteriorate. If you receive oils that have been shipped in plastic or clear glass, you should immediately transfer the essential oils to dark colored glass bottles upon arrival, unless you are going to be using all of the essential oil up within a week.

- It's a smart idea to keep empty bottles on hand. If you are buying from a supplier that ships in plastic, you should ask them how long the oil has been stored in the plastic bottles prior it being shipped. It's best if you can buy from suppliers that transfer their essential oils to plastic just before they ship.

- Some suppliers or vendors also sell larger quantities of oil in aluminum bottles. If the inside of the bottle is lined, aluminum is acceptable.

- You should avoid purchasing essential oils that have a rubber eyedropper bulb in the top because the essential oil could dissolve the rubber dropper and that would cause contamination to the oil.

- Look for vendors that promote that they test all their oils that supply samples that you can try before you buy, and that give you confidence in their knowledge by providing in-depth information on each of their essential oils and that provide other aromatherapy information that builds confidence.

- If you are comparing online vendors, start by sending out an e-mail to each of them with a list of questions that you have. This is a great way to discover just how helpful they are and how much knowledgeable they have.

- Be cautious of vendors that sell all of their essential oils for the same price. This doesn't automatically mean that their oils are not pure or of good quality, but it can. Some oils, like Rose, Neroli and Jasmine to name just a few, should cost considerably more than say ylang ylang or geranium. A high quality patchouli should cost more than eucalyptus. The basic citrus oils like lemon or sweet orange oils are the least expensive oils.

- When you buy essential oils locally, watch for oils that have dust on the top of the bottles. This indicates that the 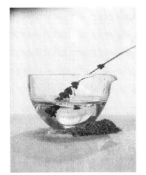 essential oils have been sitting there for some time. Over time, most essential oils will oxidize, which also means they will lose their therapeutic properties, and their aroma will also diminish.

The bottle you buy should be sealed so that the oil does not become contaminated. Make sure that the store has their essential oil tester bottles available so that you can sample the essential oils.

- If you are buying from a catalog or web site look for sites that list both the common essential oil's name and their botanical name (Latin name), the method of extraction and the country of origin. If this information isn't provided then contact them to see if they can provide this information. For example, there are numerous varieties of Cedarwood, Bay, Chamomile, Eucalyptus, etc., and each will have different therapeutic properties. The country of origin for the essential oils is also important because the soil conditions and climate can affect the essential oil's properties.

For example, is that rose oil absolute or is it steam distilled? Any good aromatherapy supplier should know how important and how necessary it is to provide this 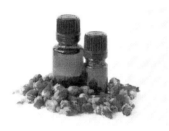 information, so if suppliers aren't providing it they are either not knowledgeable about how important it is to supply this information, they buy their oils from a variety of distributors and don't want to have to update their web site or catalogue every time they use a different source or they are just lazy.

- Educate yourself about the FDA guidelines for essential oils and aromatherapy products.

- Organic oils are typically superior to non-organic oils.

- Be careful when you buy essential oils from companies that primarily sell to the perfumery or food & beverage industries. They may have different goals in the purchase and sale of their essential oils than the goals of vendors who primarily sell oils for aromatherapy use.

The restaurant and perfumery industries desire essential oils that have a standardized aroma or flavor, so the oils sold by these sources may be redistilled to remove or add specific constituents. These adulterations or redistillations can be detrimental to the therapeutic use of the oils. Ask before you buy.

- Most of us are watching our budget, so we are tempted to buy essential oils from companies that sell them for the lowest price. While price alone does not indicate the oil quality, it can. Those vendors who spend endless hours to locate high quality oils, pay expensive fees to test the oils and provide free samples when potential customers ask, should be charging more for their oils than retailers that stock oils that they have sourced from the cheapest provider.

- When choosing to try a particular vendor, start by first placing a small first order. Your goal should be to find out if this is a vendor that you are pleased with without you wasting your money on large orders that you may not be happy with.

- Be cautious about purchasing oils from vendors at street fairs, festivals, craft shows, or other limited-time events. Many of these vendors are hobby sellers and 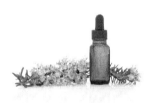 unfortunately some vendors at these events may know their customers have no recourse after the event is over. Of course, there are some highly reputable sellers at such events, but this is just a caution for those who are just beginning to buy oils and who may not yet be able to judge quality.

Organic Essential Oils

Organic essential oils are generally superior to non-organic oils. Organic oils are extracted or distilled from plants that are grown without pesticides. The therapeutic benefit and aroma of organic oils is said to be superior to oils that are non-organic

The choice is yours. You should expect to pay more for oils distilled from organic plants since it costs the provider a lot more to grow organic crops and to means maintain their land.

Tips

- Make sure that your supplies are properly cleaned. Opt for glass bowls or metal bowls as they are the most sanitary. Choose to store your body butter in glass jars.

- If you want to avoid your products becoming grainy later on leave your butters on the heat for 20 minutes to process it.

- When melting your solid oils, if you don't have a double boiler, take a Pyrex 2-Cup Measuring Cup and set it inside a pot that is filled halfway with water.

- When choosing scents for your body butter, don't be afraid to experiment. Some great options include rosemary, sweet orange, lavender, lemon and peppermint.

- Don't store your product in plastic as it breaks down and can carry toxic ingredients into your body butter and then onto your skin. Glass is your best option.

- Vitamin E won't necessarily extend the shelf life, but it will maximize the potential shelf life because it stops premature oxidization from occurring.

- If you're pregnant, you should not use essential oils.

- Crystallization occurs in vegetable butters sometimes forming tiny crystals when you heat and re-melt it. This can happen during the packaging process before you ever get it, or it can happen while you are working with it.

  Once the crystals form, the texture of the butter can become gritty. While these crystals are harmless, and will melt when they come in contact with your skin, they can detract from the appearance of your body butter. To eliminate crystals, butters need to be tempered.

- A good body butter melts when it contacts your warm skin, so you can imagine what will happen if it is exposed to the warmth of the day. That's why whipped body butters doesn't travel well. Even in your home, whipped body butters might have difficulty setting or remaining fluffy during hot days.

- Choose to use organic ingredients if you want the purest possible body butter. Some of the best prices for organic ingredients can be found online.

Conclusion

We've come to the end. At this point you know how to make very easy basic butter body recipes, you have tons of information about body butter and we've given you tons of great recipes so that you can make the best body butters you can imagine.

The rest is up to you. Have fun – be creative – try all of the recipes we offered – customize them and make them your very own!

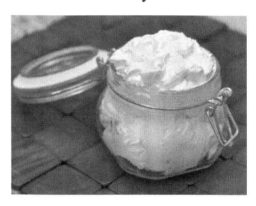

Your skin is going to love you. You'll have soft, supple skin that's healthy and sensual. You might not be off to the spa for pampering but nevertheless you're going to be pampered! Enjoy it! Keep the secret of your glowing skin to yourself or share your creations with your family and friends – you decide.

Made in the USA
Columbia, SC
06 December 2024

48625004R00076